# Sexual Problems

Herbal Remedies: Safe Alternative without Drugs

Herbal medicine has gained wide acceptance as a proven, effective health option. It has never sought to be regarded as a replacement option. Being natural, herbal medicine seeks only to provide the first stage of remedy because it is more gentle and without the side effects which chemical drugs so often induce.

In this book, a practising herbalist guides you through the many possibilities of safe home treatments, as they relate to specific health areas and problems. He covers the necessary background and provides specific recipes for you to produce your own medicines.

# Preface

The pressures and tensions of modern living have created many medical problems which, despite the constant flow of new drugs from the pharmaceutical companies, often still resist treatment. One of the more distressing of these ailments is that of sexual weakness or impotency, since our style of life in the Western World seems centred on the image of super-virility and 'machismo'.

Unfortunately, ordinary men and women rarely live up to this projected image and a sense of inadequacy and frustration can quickly set in when problems arise, particularly since of all medical conditions, help for sexual difficulties - or, the desire to gain increased virility- is one of the most difficult to obtain.

For hundreds of years herbal medicines have been known to be of help for problems such as these, and this book is aimed at helping you to find your way through the many possibilities for home treatment.

# Contents

# Introduction

An obsession with sex has become one of the most prominent features of the twentieth century. Not only have newspapers and magazines built large circulation figures by "selling sex", but sexual scenes are constantly and explicitly featured in television drama and discussed on chat shows. There has also been the establishment of sex shops, many of them selling spurious sexual aids for those who feel inadequate.

For the people of this century there has been a price to pay - in increased sexual crime, both within the family and on the street and even in "places of safety" including children's homes and medical institutions. There has also been an increase in sexually transmitted disease, although much of this has been due to the changes in sexual morality following the development of oral contraceptives, which supposedly "liberated" women, although many women are having second thoughts about this.

And the world at large faces the catastrophe of AIDS, which affects both heterosexual as well as homosexual people, and babies as well as adults.

With any revolution - social, political or religious – there will be casualties. And there have certainly been many - physical and mental - victims of the sexual revolution.

This book is not about AIDS or serious sexually transmitted diseases, or about morality. It is in response to the increasing demand noted by medical herbalists over the years from their patients for help and advice with common sexual difficulties, for which herbal medicine can be helpful. There are still many people who are too shy or embarrassed to ask for help and, in this respect, herbal medicine is useful as many remedies can be easily prepared and taken at home. This does not imply that where a serious medical condition exists that it should be treated at home from the information given in this book. In such a case the sufferer should always seek professional medical advice. However, where the pattern of the problem matches the examples given, and where the advice is applicable, then herbal treatment could well be the answer.

# Chapter 1

## Myths, Fallacies and Aphrodisiacs

Down the centuries, women seeking fertility and men desiring greater sexual potency have used aphrodisiacs and sex stimulants obtained from plants and animals.

Among the first recorded prescriptions were those of the Babylonian physicians found carved on tablets in 800BC.

Plants, such as the mandrake, orchid and sweet potato were used as sexual rejuvenates.

The mandrake, or love apple, is mentioned in the Bible, as being used by Leah to regain her fertility. Fig trees and banana trees were considered by some African tribes to be where fertility gods lived, and in India and Africa priests gave coconuts as a fertility symbol to childless women. Animal organs, including partridge brains, and the sex organs themselves have been used.

One of Africa's most fascinating animals, the rhinoceros, has become threatened with extinction because poachers shoot it to remove just one small part of its body – the horn.

This is then powdered and sold for vast sums of money in the Far East to people looking for increased virility. Research has shown, however, that it is pharmacologically inactive, any benefits being purely psychological. Flour and water would have the same effect.

While most people would say that an aphrodisiac is a remedy that creates sexual desire and heightens libido there is actually no good scientific evidence to support this concept.

In more recent times there has been an increase in illicit drugs sold on the street, such as marijuana, opiates, cocaine, and amphetamines, all of which are claimed by drug pushers to increase sexual interest and responsiveness. While it may be true that, initially, low doses may improve sexual function and interest, overuse and higher doses have the opposite effect.

Chronic marijuana use reduces sexual interest and causes impotence, cocaine and opiate addiction leads to loss of interest and performance, and overuse of amphetamines can cause psychosis with reduced sexual interest and function.

Doctors fascinated by the subject of virility have tried injecting their patients with extracts of chimpanzee sex glands, for hugely inflated fees, while one French doctor injected himself with an extract from the testes of a guinea pig. By all accounts it didn't make a significant difference.

The advent of the sex shop has led some men to believe that the simple answer to their problem is just to select an off-the-shelf magic compound. All they have to do is remember to put it on their shopping list. They are, of course, being misled, since any substance which can cause immediate involuntary erection is also likely to have serious side-effects. For example, many people may have read or heard about Spanish Fly, or Cantharides, a small beetle found in Spain, Italy, Sicily and Southern Russia, which contains a poison in its system to stop predators eating it. Dried, crushed and powdered, it has exceptionally strong irritant properties, both internally and externally. It
irritates when brought directly into contact with the skin, but if taken internally it causes inflammation, first in the stomach and then to the genital and urinary organs as it is excreted from the body. Irritation inside the ducts of the penis causes an involuntary erection. This has been its attraction to those who demand an erection at any price. However, slight miscalculations in dosage lead to extreme discomfort and even

death and, for this reason, it has been banned in most countries which have proper health regulations. Its main use was confined to causing blistering when this has been medically indicated and it was applied in a paste as a plaster. However, a remedy known as Cantharis vesicatoria (the official name of the beetle) is still manufactured by leading homœopathic chemists and available on prescription from homoeopathic physicians and practitioners, as a treatment for conditions resembling those caused by Cantharides powder.

Another so-called aphrodisiac is based on an extract fromYohimbe bark, which comes from West Africa. There is some evidence that yohimbine, an alkaloid obtained from the bark, can be beneficial to people with sexual difficulties, if it is correctly processed in a laboratory and the dose controlled. It will probably be some time in the future, however, before it will be available as a prescription medicine. Yohimbe bark, itself, can have toxic side effects and once again there is a homoeopathic remedy, Yohimbinum, which reputedly treats diseases giving a similar picture. These examples show why most of the so called aphrodisiacs in common mythology are either listed as poisons or banned from general sale. One cannot warn too strongly against the dangers of using substances which are recommended by word of mouth only. One also has to be aware of herbs that are imported into the UK from various parts of the world by private individuals. Some of these can be dangerous while others may be contaminated with drugs. There have been cases of this, particularly from India, China and the Caribbean.

It is not unknown for people to take strange and sometimes dangerous plants to medical herbalists, having imported them into the country without realising what they are. Or bottles bearing the label Spanish Fly are bought for huge sums when, in fact, they are buying a bottle of sugared water. It would be illegal, of course, to sell such a substance in the US or UK even if it were genuine.

# HERBAL TREATMENTS

An important point to be considered when dealing with sexual problems is that they rarely occur overnight. In most cases they have built up over a period of time, until the sufferer is finally driven to seek help.

With many people, the start of the problem can be caused by the illness, or death, of a partner, or perhaps an illness of their own, and to start with they are not conscious of a diminution of their sexual ability. Many have been getting steadily worse over a period of years, sometimes fifteen or twenty years, and the treatment of such cases is obviously no easy matter.

Herbal medication is unfortunately, relatively slow acting, and requires a period of time to become assimilated into the system and for the body to start showing a response. But this makes it an ideal treatment for longstanding conditions - particularly since side-effects or addiction are not generally a problem.

Later sections of this book will list recommended herbs for the treatment of sexual disorders and as tonic stimulants.

# Chapter 2

## Problems which trouble men

One of the biggest problems for the average man experiencing sexual difficulties is a lack of knowledge on the subject. While, there is no lack of reference books available which would provide many of the answers, most people are too shy or embarrassed to make the initial inquiries. Such reticence can also cause problems when the individual does decide to discuss the matter.

Unfortunately, many of the ideas that men have about sex are derived from discussions with their friends – either at school, at work or in sporting activities. Needless to say much of the information owes most of its truth to rumour and gossip!

Overcoming natural barriers, even to speak to a consultant, can often take a great deal of courage, but experience has shown that once the move has been made the questions that will be asked are often far removed from the actually difficulty which the person has come to discuss. For this reason this chapter includes the answers to some of the more common questions about sexual problems.

## ABSTINENCE

Long periods of sexual abstinence following the termination of a relationship can lead to erectile dysfunction in the male. This is frequently referred to as 'widower's syndrome', which is often a particular problem with older men and those where circumstances prevent them from enjoying sexual relations with their marital partner.

Under these circumstances, the body can best be likened to a piece of machinery - it is likely to run more smoothly when used regularly. Abstinence can lead to a slowing of the body's physical mechanisms. Also, the glandular secretions necessary for the sex act are not produced to the same requirements as when sex is regular.

Apart from the loss of these functions, abstinence probably does no particular harm to the system, as is readily demonstrated by the health and activity of the priests and monks throughout the ages who have voluntarily practised self-restraint.

The difficulty for the normal person is that when circumstances do change, it can be difficult to restart regular activity, and it can be particularly hard to break down the psychological block which tends to set up after a long abstinence. Even regular masturbation during the time that no partner is available can still lead to a sense of worry over possible failure when a partner is again available.

## SEX AND THE ELDERLY

Some people still believe that it is in some way harmful for elderly people to engage in sexual activity. But given reasonable health and no history of high blood pressure, or heart conditions, there is no reason why sexual intercourse should not be enjoyed well into old age. Indeed, it is thought to help prolong a healthy life.

Unfortunately, this is not always accepted. Society still seems to equate sexual inadequacy with ageing and rather expects the elderly not to be fully operational. Many old people may feel guilty if they are sexually active and may even succumb to being "sexless" because society expects it. Although we may not expect elderly people to climb mountains, loss of sexual desire and function is often considered to be just a step away from death.

Medical and scientific studies, starting with Kinsey in the late 1940s, on sexual behaviour in the human male and female revealed that sexual interest and activity may continue in those over the age of 90 - and even after the ninth decade.

## FREQUENCY OF EJACULATIONS

If you listen to a group of men gossiping it would be easy to imagine that the average man can perform the sexual act at least four or five times nightly, 365 days a year! While the law of possibilities may make some men capable of such a performance, Mr Average will be satisfied with a much lower performance level.

Obviously, a younger man is likely to have a higher frequency of intercourse and ejaculation in a given period than an older man. A young man in his prime could probably be capable of two to three orgasms over a two to three hour period; a middle-aged to elderly person would probably be able to average only one act of orgasm, often with a few days break in between, since the body takes much longer to recover, the older you get.

## FREQUENCY OF SEXUAL INTERCOURSE

The sexual capacity of individuals differs widely, and in some ways it is wrong to try to set down an average which could perhaps set unattainable levels for some couples. Basically, the act of making love should be as often as is right for the individuals and what may be considered correct for one couple may be totally unsuitable for another.

However, the following average statistics compiled from many years of consultations may be interesting as a comparison guide. All couples are assumed to enjoy good health, to be compatible and to have average sexual appetites.

| Age of couple | Number of acts of intercourse in week |
|---|---|
| 18-24 | 5-9 |
| 24-30 | 5-7 |
| 30-35 | 4-5 |
| 35-45 | 3-4 |
| 45-55 | 2-4 |
| 55-60 | 2-3 |
| 60-65 | 2 |
| over 65 | 1 |

Six out of ten married couples, aged between 60 and 74, remain sexually active, compared with three out of ten aged over 75. Although sexual interest and activity may decrease as people get older, giving up sex altogether is usually due to a decline in the physical health of either or both of the partners.

Impotency, even in men aged between 80 and 90, has been found to be due more often to psychological than physical causes.

Sexually active men aged over 65 have intercourse about four times a month, compared with two or three times a week in the fifties and five or more times a week for young newly-marrieds.

Unlike oestrogen in women, the male hormone, testosterone, continues to be produced well into old age, but the amount is often insufficient and changes take place in the genital organs. The testicles begin to atrophy and become softer, while the prostate gland becomes larger. Less semen is produced and ejaculation is less forceful. Older women who are in good health and have an available partner are able to enjoy sexual relations until very old age. According to Masters and johnson whose work on human sexuality caused a storm in the 1960s "there is no time limit drawn by advancing years to female sexuality".

It is mainly myths about the menopause, which decree that being post-menopausal means an end to sexual desire and attractiveness, which so often leads to depression and other psychological illnesses.

Although there are physiological and physical changes in the older woman, such as a decrease in vaginal lubrication, thinning of the vaginal mucosa, reduction in size of the clitoris and loss of breast firmness, there is no evidence of any significant loss in clitoral sensation. But some women, as a result of hormonal deprivation, do find intercourse painful, due to deficient lubrication or to uterine contractions during orgasm. The bladder and urethra are also more susceptible to symptoms of cystitis, such as burning and irritation. These conditions are amenable to treatment.

## MASTURBATION

Kinsey reported in 1953 that 93 per cent of men and 58 per cent of women interviewed reported that they had masturbated at some time in their lives. He added that about one-third of the women who said they had never masturbated before marriage, or whose masturbation had never led to an orgasm, did not reach orgasm during intercourse with their partners in the first year of marriage.
Most of these women also reported that they had not had an orgasm during the first five years of marriage.

Modern thinking about masturbation is quite different from the condemning attitude of the Victorians. It is now considered to be a natural practice, neither harmful nor weakening, unless carried to excess. Indeed, masturbation therapy is sometimes used by sex therapists in the treatment of patients who complain of being an orgasmic.

Zoologists have pointed out that masturbation also occurs naturally among the primates, even when there is ample opportunity for copulation. As in humans, a higher percentage of male animals than females masturbate. It has been observed in various species, including female dogs, rats, elephants, porcupines, chinchillas and dolphins.

Myths about masturbation have been perpetuated, however. In the mid-1970s a survey of medical students revealed that one in six believed there was a link between masturbation and mental illness.

But statements by religious leaders have not helped to clear the confusion inherited from the past. For example, Pope Paul VI, in 1966, described masturbation as "an intrinsically and seriously disordered act". The modern medical view is that it is only damaging if indulged in persistently.

## NOCTURNAL ERECTIONS

Penile erections in the male during sleep are a naturally occurring phenomenon. They are important to the medical investigator for, if erections, or tumescence, occur during sleep in a man complaining of impotence it reveals that the cause of his problem is psychogenic rather than physical.

Normal men of various ages have between three and five periods of penile tumescence lasting from 27 to 38 minutes each during sleep at night. Conversely, impotent men suffering from diseases such as diabetes, serious kidney disease, alcoholism or injuries to the spinal cord, have less tumescence. When erection does occur it is also for a shorter time.

Most nocturnal erections occur during REM, or the rapid eye movement phase of sleep. This is when the eyes undergo rapid, jerky movements associated with dreaming and with an increased heart and respiration rate. Penile tumescence is not confined to adult men. It was first considered to be a sleep phenomenon of male babies, but in 1944 researchers observed the same occurrence in adults. It is now realised that it occurs in males from birth to old age. Normal elderly men have three or four erections a night, lasting for about one-fifth of their total sleeping time. Morning erections are similar to those during the night.

It used to be commonly believed that they were caused by the presence of a full bladder, but this has been disproved.

## SPONTANEOUS EJACULATION

Ejaculation is usually associated with sexual intercourse or genital stimulation as a result of masturbation, but it can also occur spontaneously during sleep when it is known as a nocturnal emission or a "wet dream". Four out of five men have experienced nocturnal emissions at some time during their lives, usually during early adulthood.

The emissions are usually explained as being due to "psychic stimulation". Subconscious fantasies, if intense, trigger off the orgasm, which is considered to be a natural and healthy automatic release of abundant supplies of seminal fluid. It has been observed that nocturnal emissions become less frequent after marriage and where there is regular sexual activity.

Some men who have nocturnal emissions are unable to ejaculate during normal intercourse despite being fertile and able to attain and hold an erection. One investigator reported that these patients seem to produce excessive saliva in the mouth instead of ejaculating.

The ancient Greeks believed that "wet dreams" were due to the oral attentions of evil female spirits. It became the custom to spread crushed onion leaves around the bed of single men to deter them.

## HOMOSEXUAL FIXATION

Many men worry unnecessarily that they may be homosexual. This can arise when a sexual problem occurs and may be exacerbated by them thinking back to their schooldays when they may have had a "crush" on a male friend. But during pre-puberty and puberty boys often have a fixation on male friends of a similar age. This is not usually regarded as homosexual behaviour, since as the boy grows older, his interest changes to the opposite sex.

The best course for the adult male who has such a worry is to seek the help of a counsellor who is trained to deal with such problems.

## PRIAPISM

This is a condition in which there is a persistent, usually painful erection of the penis. The name is derived from Priapus, the Roman god of male sexuality and fertility. Priapism is relatively rare, but it can afflict men of all age groups. Although it may be associated with sexual activity it is not necessarily induced by sexual desire or stimulation.

Among the known causes are various medicines and drugs, including aphrodisiacs containing yohimbin, cantharides, androgens and strychnine. Marijuana and alcohol have been implicated and also drugs used to treat blood pressure, including guanethidine, hydralazine and prazosin. But in about half the cases there is no apparent causative factor. In nearly a third of cases in adult men and in the majority of cases among boys the condition is associated with sickle cell anaemia. But to put matters in perspective it should be emphasised that although sickle cell disease is the second most common cause of priapism in the adult, priapism occurs in less than four per cent of sickle cell cases. Unfortunately, in these adults repeated attacks of priapism can lead to impotence.

There are many other causes of priapism with as many different treatments, Homoeopaths would, no doubt, think of using cantharides, while herbalists would normally use an infusion of a sexual sedative, such as black willow bark in their treatment.

## PENIS SIZE

This is a perennial subject for discussion and speculation, and probably one about which there are more misunderstandings than any other.

Basically, there are two types of penis. The first is relatively small when at the rest position, but under stimulation becomes hard and can more than double in size. The second is a naturally long type of penis which, when stimulated, may increase in size by only two to five centimetres (one or two inches) and, in many cases, not even this.

The dimensions of the average erect Caucasian male penis are approximately 16.5 centimetres (61/2 inches) in length and approximately 11 centimetres (41/2 inches) in circumference; while at rest it may average 6 to 9 centimetres (21f2 to 31f2 inches). The average of the slacker type of penis may be 10 to 13 centimetres (4 to 5 inches) at rest and 15 to 18 centimetres (6 to 7 inches) when erect.

It is, in fact, not the size of the penis but the technique of coition which ensures mutual bodily enjoyment between partners.

## SOME COMMON OBSTACLES TO SATISFACTORY SEXUAL RELATIONS

### OBESITY

This diminishes virility and saps strength and energy. The remedy is simple – lose weight and take more exercise. Re-examine your food intake and change to a better diet with fewer calories, less fat and sugar, more fresh fruit and vegetables and more fibre. Gradually increase the amount of exercise you take; walking and swimming are good ways to take gentle exercise at first.

### NERVOUS TENSION AND NERVOUS DEBILI1Y

Tension can quickly diminish sexual performance even to the point of impotency. Weakness is often exacerbated by stomach disorders and persistent flatulence.

## RESPIRATORY PROBLEMS

Serious chest problems progressively weaken the physique and thus make sexual activity difficult.

## DOMESTIC DISCORD

Excessive tension caused by arguments or problems with a partner or among members of the family can cause sexual problems.

## ALCOHOLIC STIMUIATION

Spirits considerably diminish sexual performance – and beers do nothing to help either! There is no doubt about the truth of this - partial intoxication inhibits and dulls sexual enjoyment; chronic alcoholics are usually impotent.

## PROSTATE GLAND

This important gland produces most of the fluid in the semen. Disease of the prostate is almost inevitable in the older man - the longer a man lives the more likely he is to suffer from prostate trouble.

The gland, which lies at the neck of the bladder, surrounds the urethra - the tube leading from the bladder and through the penis. In later life, as hormone function alters, the gland tends to increase in size and shape and begins to restrict the flow of urine through the urethra. The contractions of an enlarged prostate also become weaker, less seminal fluid is produced and the force of ejaculation decreases.

This benign enlargement of the prostate also produces urinary frequency, and a slower urinary flow.

With surgical removal of the prostate, the male is unable to ejaculate as the ejaculatory components are also removed. Treatment of an enlarged prostate can be undertaken with herbal medicines and nutritional supplements. A popular first-line remedy is obtained from dried pumpkin seeds. It has been observed that prostate troubles are far less frequent in countries where people regularly chew pumpkin seeds. Medical herbalists tend to combine several herbs, depending on individual symptoms and may very well include powdered pumpkin seeds, containing cucurbitacin, grown from special varieties of pumpkin.

## AN OLDER MAN WITH A YOUNG WIFE

With society shifting towards later marriages, second marriages, and non-marriage relationships, it is not unusual to see older men and women with younger partners. In most cultures it still seems to be more acceptable for the man to be older than the woman. A relationship between a young woman and a man old enough to be her father is considered more normal than the other way round, although in some countries, including Britain, Sweden and West Germany, marriages between older women and young men are rapidly increasing. The older man who marries a young woman is regarded as some kind of sex symbol. However, these liaisons can run into trouble if the man loses his confidence - impotency is not an uncommon complaint.

## COMMONLY PRACTISED METHODS OF CONTRACEPTION BY MEN

### COITUS INTERRUPTUS

The act of swiftly withdrawing the penis from the vagina immediately prior to ejaculation is not a reliable method of contraception because some semen can be emitted before orgasm and result in conception. It is extremely bad for the nerves of both partners and if practised for a lengthy period can give rise to psychological disturbances.

## INTERCOURSE TERMINATED BEFORE ORGASM

Without a natural culmination of the sex act the parties are inevitably frustrated and emotionally disturbed. This is an unsatisfactory and dangerous behaviour pattern and one which can lead to medical problems for the man.

## CONDOMS

Convenient and reliable to use, condoms also have the merit of being hygienic and permitting nearly normal intercourse. They are recommended as a method of contraception for men.

# LICE

With the increase of sexual activity outside of marriage, and particularly with the ease of modem travel, lice have again become a modem scourge - although it is strange how few men are able to recognise the symptoms.

There are three main types of lice, all of which can be caught during intercourse, but one of these, the Crab louse, is most common.

## HEAD LOUSE (PEDICULUS CAPITIS)

Eggs are usually laid behind the ears and at the back of the head, although the louse can be distributed throughout the hair. Very common also among schoolchildren.

## BODY LOUSE (PEDICULUS VESTIMENTE)

This type of louse stays mainly in the seams of under clothing, both around the lower part of the body and the upper arms. Bite marks will be visible as red irritations.

## CRAB LOUSE (PHTHIRUS PUBIS)

This one is normally found in the hairs of the pubic region in which it lays its eggs. It causes intense itching and is most likely to be spread through sexual contact. Treatment for all three of these is relatively simple and straightforward and any chemist should have suitable treatments available, including preparations containing pyrethrum.

# Chapter 3

## Sexual difficulties common to adult men

The great majority of failures and difficulties experienced during the attempted act of intercourse are usually related in one form or another to nervous tension and psychological inhibitions. Probably in only a small number of cases is there organic disease present.

## PREMATURE EJACULATION

There appear to be a number of definitions of premature ejaculation, ranging from a stopwatch definition, such as ejaculation after less than 30 seconds of intercourse, to a performance definition - less than 10 penile thrusts. But there are other more vague definitions, including one that describes premature ejaculation as a condition in which a man arrives at orgasm and ejaculation "before he desires to do so".

Most people would probably agree that premature ejaculation is best described as spontaneous ejaculation and orgasm immediately before, or immediately after penetration, and occurring before it was desired. The time factor seems to be important as studies by sex therapists show that normal intercourse for most couples appears to last between four and seven minutes. This is the time required for most women to achieve orgasm. Many women have reported that they are able to achieve orgasm in less than a minute.

Premature ejaculation is more likely to occur in men early in a relationship and most cases can be expected to resolve spontaneously as the flame of passion begins to cool. But repeated failure to effect a normal intercourse in a man who is anxious or over-excited can give rise to a conditioned reflex which persistently trigger soft ejaculation. It can also occur to the man whose wife suffers from vaginismus.

Some men who complain of premature ejaculation are married to assertive women and have difficulty in expressing their own anger. The condition can become a way of gaining control over the relationship.

Treatment may be successful with herbal anaphrodisiacs which reduce sexual excitement, but psychotherapy may also be indicated.

## IMPOTENCY

A number of diseases and drugs have been linked with impotency. Among the most well known are high blood pressure, diabetes mellitus and cardiovascular disease - particularly angina, and anxiety following a heart attack - infections of the prostate and skin of the penis, neurological diseases, including multiple sclerosis, Parkinson's disease and spinal cord injuries.

As well as prescribed drugs, alcohol, marijuana and narcotics can also cause impotence. Among prescribed drugs, some for treatment of blood pressure are common offenders and, indeed, are one of the reasons why patients fail to comply with the physician's treatment. If they can be discontinued the body generally restores itself. It is difficult to establish just how many drugs do cause impotency as a side effect. Even the prescribing doctors are not always aware of the potential problem. But there are probably 40 or 50 drugs in regular use which have this side effect and it is quite wrong that they should be administered to a patient without him being told of the possible effects as, even if the condition restores itself, there can be a psychological end result.

## SEX URGE BUT NO ERECTION

The sexual desires of the subject are normal- in fact often excessive - sometimes heightened by erotic fantasies and visual stimulation, but erection is not achieved and intercourse is not possible. The most frequent cause of this distressing condition is psychological inhibitions, guilt complexes and feelings of inadequacy. Severe nervous tension and loss of confidence are often contributory factors.

## SEX URGE BUT WEAK ERECTION

Some men can experience a sex urge but the penis remains too limp to permit vaginal penetration, or they may experience a weak erection that soon becomes limp or flaccid. This is a similar condition to 'Sex urge but no erection'. Continuation of the weakness occasions strong psychological inhibitions and expectations of failure; fixation is thus established and a mental block prevents normal intercourse.

## SEX URGE AND LIMP ERECTION BUT NO ORGASM

This is a further variation of the previous two conditions that frequently gives rise to marital discord and discontent.

## NO SEX URGE, DESIRE OR ERECTION

This condition is infrequent, and if the sufferer has no organic disease is probably due to longstanding guilt complexes and nervous debility.

## INFERTILITY

Generally, sexual relations will be quite normal until it is discovered that the wife is not conceiving when a baby is desired. Problems of gaining erection and ejaculation can however quickly arise due to guilt feelings, even though the man may not be the infertile partner.

## SOLVING THE PROBLEMS

All of these distressing inadequacies can be greatly relieved, provided the sufferer will give his understanding co-operation to his adviser or follow a sensible course of treatment. Just as a car can be tuned to give greater performance, so can a man be helped to adequate sexual ability. The case histories in the next chapter will give some guidelines to possible treatments.

# Chapter 4

## Case histories

The following examples are given to show the variety and complications which can arise in a person's sexual life, and they illustrate some of the problems discussed in the previous chapter. Suitable herbs can be selected from the later chapter 'Some Recommended Herbs', choosing those which conform with the recommendations shown. Obviously details of individuals have been changed to prevent any recognition, since complete confidentiality must always be maintained.

## CASE HISTORY 1

MR P.M.
Age 25 years.

Occupation- Company representative.
Problem-Mr P.M. asked for help in maintaining his virility, since his job took him to many different parts of the country and he found this exhausting both physically and sexually.
Conclusion- Over-indulgence.

Recommended- treatment Vitamin E, ginseng, herbal tonic stimulants.

Result- After a two-month course of treatment, he reported by telephone that he felt his old self and did not need to continue with the recommendations.

## CASE HISTORY 2

MR AH.C AND MRSM.LC
Age - 47 years and 45 years.

Occupations - The husband and wife were proprietors of a small hotel on the coast.
Problem During consultation it became clear that the gross takings of the business were insufficient to enable enough staffto be employed. MrAH.C complained that he suffered intermittent severe flatulence and indigestion, felt tense and always'on edge', and often felt 'weak and shaky'. Although he slept well, he awakened 'tired and dull'. He stated that although he thought a lot about sex and desired it, he did not have an erection. When he did attempt intercourse his penis was tumescent, but limp, and after vaginal penetration it became

soft and he was unable to ejaculate. He was very worried and depressed.

Mrs M.LC complained that she suffered bad insomnia, sleeping only 2 to 3 hours a night. She was also troubled with severe migraine and pains across the shoulders, and fitsof depression with crying spells. Hair was dry and brittle and complexion rough and dark around the eyes. Said she did not care about sex now but would alwaysdo it for her husband. She did not worry about her husband's sexual difficulties because she thought they were 'getting past it now'.

Conclusion Both were suffering from acute nervous tension occasioned by overwork and monotony. Also Mrs M.LC was entering her menopause.

Recommended treatment - A high protein diet avoiding high acid concentration foods such as citrus juices, salads and greens. Cut down on consumption of drinks such as tea and coffee which have concentrations of caffeine. Take small but frequent meals.

Mr AH.C to take herbal nerve tonics, tonic stimulants and a course of ginseng.

Mrs M.LC to take herbal nerve tonics, Avena and St John's Wort to assist menopausal symptoms.

Results - Interviewed two months later, Mr AH.C stated that they were feeling very much better and Mrs M.I.C was sleeping well and looking younger and fresher. They were having sex two or three times a week. He was able to achieve a full erection, often involuntary, and his wife was now eager and co-operative for sexual intercourse.

## CASE HISTORY 3
MR CH.
Age 64 years.

Occupation Retired.

Problem – Mr CH. stated that after six years as a widower he had married again to a lady of 35 years, a divorcee. He complained that he felt 'run down' and that his wife did not understand him. She was willing to have sex every night but she was bad tempered and impatient when he could not accommodate her. His penis only half erected and a weak ejaculation, without sensation, occurred before full entry. He was not capable of the sex act more than twice a week, although he had regularly masturbated during his years alone.

Conclusion He was troubled by a loss of confidence and a guilt complex, as well as an unwarranted physical inferiority fixation.

Recommended treatment - Tonic stimulants and a nerve tonic.

Result - After four weeks, Mr CH. reported that he was more able to maintain a full erection and was accomplishing normal intercourse. He was also experiencing sensation again at orgasm, felt more confident, and was getting on much better with his wife.

# Chapter 5

## Sexual difficulties common to adult women

The sexual problems which can afflict women are also very often of psychological origin. The following are the main types of problems which women are most likely to experience in everyday life.

### FAILURE TO ACHIEVE ORGASM

This is the most common complaint among women. There has been such an overwhelming preoccupation with it by women's magazines that it has become a source of anxiety and distress, not only among women who feel abnormal if they do not experience it, but also among men who feel dissatisfied if they cannot bring their partner to a climax.

Many women do not achieve orgasm during intercourse, simply because the male ejaculates too soon. They may very well be able to experience orgasm by masturbation, or by a combination of manual stimulation and intercourse, or by the use of sex aids, but they may worry that a method they find successful is not the way it should be done. Orgasm itself may vary in degree of intensity and may occur on some occasions and not on others. Failure to achieve orgasm by any method is more likely to be due to emotional than physical problems and may be helped by counselling. In some cases it is due to sexual abuse in childhood. Frequently, it is due to the inability to relax.

### LACK OF DESIRE

Lack of interest in sexual activity can be due to domestic discord, wavering affection or health problems. The woman may be disgruntled with her partner or may be averse to all sexual fantasy and feeling. Lack of desire is also a symptom of nervous tension or to physical exhaustion from overwork. Many women suffer through being involved in business affairs as well as running a home and bringing up a family. A wavering libido should be regarded as an early warning sign.

Women with a number of small children find that everyday domestic chores wear them down or are so monotonous that they become sexually debilitated and are unable to take any interest in their partner's sexual demands. A change in domestic responsibilities, more emphasis on leisure pursuits and a good herbal tonic can be very beneficial.

## LACK OF AROUSAL

This may be associated with lack of desire, but is often due to faulty technique. With sexual arousal there is vaginal lubrication, nipple erection and breast engorgement. Even when a women desires sexual intercourse she may find that arousal does not occur and may feel there is something wrong with her. If her partner 'is desirable' and sexual technique is not at fault, the problem may be due to an internal emotional conflict requiring psychotherapy.

## PAINFUL INTERCOURSE

The medical term for this is dyspareunia. It is one of the more common sexual complaints and affects women of all ages. It can be caused by both physical and psychological factors. About one in five of all women seeking a gynaecological consultation do so because of dyspareunia. A small percentage of these women may be referred for psychotherapy. The site of pain varies. It may be felt at the vaginal entrance or deep inside at the cervix.

Most women experiencing painful intercourse suffer from vaginitis due to infections of the genital tract, or to pelvic disease, such as endometriosis. But pain can also be due to a tumour, a possibility which should not be overlooked.

The next most common cause occurs in post-menopausal women and is associated with lack of lubrication of the vagina due to a fall in oestrogen levels. Dyspareunia due to lack of lubrication also affects women whose husbands suffer from either premature ejaculation and attempt penetration too early, or from retarded ejaculation, leading to prolonged sexual intercourse with damage to the vaginal lining.

A number of other conditions, including allergies, glandular infections and postnatal conditions, such as scarring, can also cause pain.

Among the psychological factors inducing dyspareunia are those which also lead to failure of orgasm. Sexual abuse in childhood, phobias and depression can all be triggering factors - painful intercourse can be due to a painful relationship.

## VAGINISMUS

Some women have such an extreme distaste for intercourse that they refuse all attempts at penetration by their partners. They may experience vaginismus, a painful spasm of the vaginal muscles, which tightly closes the entrance to the vaginal canal, making intercourse impossible. The condition can also occur when sexual intercourse is imagined or feared. It may be due to painful sexual experiences in the past. Often, the woman does not associate the pain with her inner feelings because the vaginismus has become a conditioned response. She may even be desperate to have a baby and cannot understand why she is suffering so much pain. In some cases the woman is sexually interested and can be sexually aroused, but will experience spasm just before penetration.

Untreated, the condition can be disastrous for a marriage. The woman may be rejected by her partner, or the partner may suffer impotence. Treatment is usually by a combination of techniques, including relaxation, special exercises, herbal nervines and relaxants, and counselling in sexual techniques designed to allow the woman to control penetration by her partner. The success rate of treatment is particularly good.

## THE AVOIDANCE OF MUNDANE ROUTINE SEX

A woman should never be taken for granted - she should be vital and surprising and never dull and obsessed with routine household affairs. Sex enters a thrilling new dimension when it surprises - and can afford even the most matter-of-fact husband delightful titillation when it is quite unexpected and taking place in unfamiliar surroundings. Take the initiative and be at your best.

## VAGINITIS

Inflammation of the vagina is a common cause of women seeking treatment. It often produces symptoms similar to cystitis and a misdiagnosis may have been made. Sometimes the condition may be due to a sexually transmitted disease. Such infections need proper treatment as they can lead to other conditions, such as infertility, or endometritis.

The main symptoms of vaginitis, are itching, discharge and painful urination.

When the condition is due to an infection, the woman has to be careful that cross-infeciton with her partner does not occur. This factor is often forgotten and is the reason why many infections keep recurring. During treatment for vaginal infection it is paramount that the woman either avoids sexual intercourse, or that her partner uses a sheath.

Most infections are associated with Candida albicans or Trichomonas uaginalis. The discharge due to Candida is thick and white, rather like cottage cheese; with Trichomonas it is a yellowy-green, and frothy, and has an unpleasant smell.

Trichomonas is commonly found in the normal healthy vagina. It is only when the population level of the organism has increased to above normal levels that 'an infection' is said to have occurred. It can also be found in the normal prostate. Changes in the vagina's acidity levels may trigger the multiplication of Trichomonas, which causes irritation, with itching and burning, ranging from slight and short lived to prolonged and very upsetting.

Likewise, Candida is a normal inhabitant of the mouth and bowel. When Candida 'infects' the mouth it is known as thrush or oral monoliasis. It is common in newborn babies whose mothers have Candida vaginitis. Candidosis has become an epidemic due to the advent of oral contraceptives and the overuse of antibiotics and steroid drugs.

Antibiotics suppress the varieties of bacteria in the body that normally hold Candida in check. Fortunately, live yoghurt contains bacteria which inhibit Candida and, therefore, a popular first-line treatment for Candida infection is to eat plenty of yoghurt and to use it locally as a cream.

Vaginitis in women after the menopause and in those who have had their ovaries removed is usually due to oestrogen deficiency. The lining of the vagina becomes thinner and drier, giving rise to surface damage during intercourse. Infection and inflammation may then ensue. Hormone creams containing oestrogen are popularly prescribed by physicians, although a vitamin E cream, dietary treatment and oestrogenic herbal medicines are often successful.

Garlic,liquorice, marigold, goldenseal, barberry, tea tree oil, fennel, alfalfa and red clover are among the herbal agents that can be used to clear up most vaginal infections. Garlic is antifungal, antibiotic and antiviral; liquorice is antiviral and oestrogenic; marigold is antiseptic and oestrogenic; fennel is diuretic and oestrogenic; red clover is a blood purifier and oestrogenic; goldenseal and barberry are antiseptic and antibacterial; and tea tree oil is antifungal and antibacterial. In resistant cases professional advice is called for.

Vaginitis in young girls is often due to organisms from the nose or mouth being introduced innocently into the vagina by the girl's unwashed hands. Candida infection is commonly found, as prior to menstruation, oestrogen, which alters the vaginal environment, is not produced.

# Chapter 6

## More case histories

These case histories will be of general interest in illustrating some of the female problems outlined in the previous chapter.

### CASE HISTORY 4

MRS M.HO.
Age 36 years.

Occupation - Secretary.

Problem - She explained that until her mother died she had been a virgin. She then married an ex-soldier older than herself and of a different religion. She complained that she could not have any sexual relations with her husband and that he was now asking her to leave home. This made her very tense and depressed.

Conclusion - She was suffering from vaginismus (involuntary total frigidity) and strong psychological inhibitions. Recommended treatment A course of ginseng and herbal nerve tonics.

Result - A month later she reported that she had accomplished fullcoitus with her husband and was feeling more settled.

### CASE HISTORY 5

MRS KO.
Age 26 years.
Occupation Housewife.

Problem - Mrs KO. asked for help on behalf of her husband who, after a medical examination, was found to have a very low sperm count. They had been unable to conceive and this was putting strong pressures on their marriage.
Conclusion Both husband and wife needed some assistance both to encourage conception and to reduce stress.

Recommended treatment - For Mr KO., Vitamin E and ginseng. For Mrs KO., herbal nerve tonics and ginseng.

Results - Mrs KO. reported that her husband's sperm count had greatly improved and that while she had still not conceived, there were more relaxed about the situation and hopeful for the future.

# Chapter 7

## Drugs related to sexual disorders

A number of commonly used drugs are associated with sexual dysfunction. Houseleek Perhaps the most important is alcohol.

## ALCOHOL

The effect that drinking alcohol has on sexual performance varies according to the quantity taken. In some people small amounts of alcohol may actually improve performance because it reduces inhibition. Larger quantities, however, have a sedating effect and, in men, interfere with the ability to gain an erection. Indeed, many regular drinkers report an increased sexual desire but an inability to perform.

Studies have shown that alcohol interferes with the metabolism of the male hormone, testosterone. Regular male drinkers have been shown to have a reduced blood level of the hormone. Unfortunately, a man who drinks and is experiencing sexual difficulties is likely to take solace by drinking even more so entering into a vicious circle.

Alcohol has been described as the most commonly available contraceptive and it is likely that it is the major cause of impotence and sterility in the UK.

## ANTIHYPERTENSIVE

Drugs used to treat blood pressure are a common cause of sexual disorder in men. It is surprising the number of men seen by medical herbalists who have been prescribed blood pressure drugs and who complain of reduced virility, but who are unaware of the association. Obviously, they have not been told of the risk by their doctors. But as blood pressure is more common in the older man it would not be surprising if he did not assume incorrectly that his reduced virility was to do with his age, rather than his drugs. One wonders how many couples are suffering needlessly when alternative drugs or natural treatments could be used.

Blood pressure drugs that can induce sexual dysfunction include:

| Name | Class of drug | Adverse effect |
| --- | --- | --- |
| CARACEPLUS lisinopril and hydrochlorothiazide | ACE inhibitor and diuretic | Impotence |
| DECLINAX Debrisoquine sulphate | Adrenergic neurone blocker | ejaculation failure |
| DIBENYLINE Phenoxybenzamine hydrochloride | Vasodilator | ejaculation failure |
| ESBATAL Bethanidine sulphate | Adrenergic neurone blocker | ejaculation failure |
| INNOZIDE enalapril maleate and hydrochlorothiazide | ACE inhibitor and diuretic | impotence |
| ISMELIN Guanethidine sulphate | Adrenergic neurone blocker | ejaculation failure |

Antidepressant drugs may also cause sexual disturbances, particularly those classified as tricyclic antidepressants and monoamine oxidase inhibitors.

# Chapter 8

## Herbal treatments and medication

The formulae that follow are all suitable to make up as directed, following the given instructions and using quantities shown as percentages of the whole. Ingredients should be available from herbal shops, herbalists and many health food shops - if any difficulty is experienced consult the list of suppliers at the back of the book.

## INFORMATION ON THE PREPARATION OF HERBS

### DECOCTIONS

The herbs are cut, ground up or bruised and covered with cold fresh water. This mixture is then boiled for up to half an hour, allowed to cool and then strained through a fine mesh. Allow 28 grams of the herbs to 568 ml of water (1 Oz to 1 pint). This method is normally used when the herb is unsuitable to make as an infusion. The usual dose is from one to two fluid ounces three times daily.

### INFUSIONS

Tea is made by the process of infusion. Prepare the herbs to be used and quickly pour boiling water on them. Allow the mixture to stand for about half an hour, stirring frequently and when ready strain off the liquid.Allow28 grams of herbs to 568 ml of water (1 oz to 1 pint). The usual dose is one or two fluid ounces three times daily, usually one after each main meal.

## SOLID EXTRACTS

Start with a strong infusion of the herbs required and evaporate over low heat until a heavy consistency is obtained.

## TINCTURES

This process is used for herbs and drugs which become useless when heated, or for those herbs which are not amenable to treatment by water.

The tinctures prescribed by medical herbalists are made commercially with pure alcohol for which a government licence is necessary.

They may also undergo the process of maceration and filtration several times in order to strengthen the tincture and to reduce the final alcohol content to a minimum.

For home use tinctures can be made with pure or diluted brandy, but this is a rather expensive process. However, the preparation can be much stronger than a simple infusion or decoction, the ratio ranging from 1:5 - one ounce of the herb to five fluid ounces of menstruum, up to 1:20 – one ounce of herb to 20 fluid ounces of brandy.

Most tinctures need a 25 per cent proportion of alcohol to water. Dosage ranges from 10 drops to a teaspoonful in water depending on the strength of the main ingredient. The advantage of tinctures is that they are more convenient to use and they keep well.

## ESSENTIAL OILS

Pure oils extracted from plants are extremely potent – and toxic in overdose - and should not be taken internally without adequate knowledge of the individual remedy.

One or two drops of the oil, shaken in water, at most forms a single dose. One drop of undiluted peppermint oil dropped on to the tongue, for example, is so strong it makes the eyes water. The potency of essential oils can be seen from the affect of just adding a few drops into bath water. For home use this is the recommended way of using these oils. The properties of the oils, research has shown, is absorbed into the body via the skin. Prescribed correctly, plant oils are a useful addition to the herbal dispensary.

## SOME SIMPLE FORMULAE TO MAKE AT HOME

### A GOOD GENERAL TONIC

Kola 1 part
Damiana 5 parts
Saw Palmetto 1 part

Make up as an infusion

### A SEXUAL STIMULANT TONIC

Ginseng - 1 part
Kola - 1 part
Damiana - 4 parts
Saw Palmetto - 1 part

Make up as an infusion.

Damiana 65%
Saw Palmetto 10%
Quercus 5%
Ginseng 5%
Tincture of Ginger 5%
Tincture of Gentian 5%

Make up Damiana, Saw Palmetto, Quercus and Ginseng as a decoction. Add the two tinctures. Take one fluid ounce two or three times daily.

# Chapter 9

## Some recommended herbs

This section of the book lists in alphabetical order some of the herbs which can be used in the treatment of conditions mentioned earlier, together with other herbs of a generally beneficial nature.

### Alfalfa
MED/GAGO SATIVA

Also known as - Lucerne.

Found wild - Europe.

Appearance - Similar to a large clover

Parts used - Leaves and stem.

Therapeutic uses - Alfalfais rich in minerals and contains enzymes which aid the assimilation of nutrients into the blood. It thus has a reputation as a body builder and is ideal for those who seek to increase their weight. It has been used traditionally as a method of increasing the size of the breasts. It also improves milk production in nursing mothers and is indicated in the treatment of prostatitis.

### Amaranth
AMARANTHUS HYPOCHONDRIACUS

Also known as - Love Lies Bleeding.

Found wild - UK and Europe.

Appearance - A common garden plant with crimson flowers similar to a cockscomb.

Part used - Herb.

Therapeutic uses - Treatment of diarrhoea and menorrhagia. As an astringent. Helpful in all cases of looseness of the bowel.

Prepared as - Decoction.

### American White Pond Lily
NYMPHAE ODORATA

Also known as Water Cabbage.

Found wild United States.

Appearance Perennial aquatic herb with large white flowers.

Parts used - Root and leaves.

Therapeutic uses - Antiseptic an  soothing astringent indicated for the treatment of weakness of the pelvic organs, simple vaginal discharge, laxity of vaginal tissue, inflammation of prostate, cervical ulcerations and lesions.

Prepared as - Powder, decoction, infusion, lotion, douche, poultice, fluid extract, tincture.

### Arenaria Rubra
LEPIGONUM RUBRUM

Also known as Sandwort.

Found wild - Malta and Corsica.

Appearance A small low growing plant with small pink flowers. Part used - Herb.

Therapeutic uses - Diuretic. Of great value for the treatment of cystitis and stones. Also for bladder complaints.

Prepared as - Infusion.

### Arbutus, Trailing
EPIGAEA REPENS

Also known as - Mayflower, Ground Laurel.

Found wild - North America.

Appearance - Procumbent herb, evergreen leaves and white or pink, fragrant flowers.

Part used - Herb.

Therapeutic uses - A diuretic. Most effective for urinary disorders. Also has astringent properties.

Prepared as - Infusion.


## Arrach
CHENOPODIUM OLIDUM

Found wild - Throughout Europe.

Appearance - Small inconspicuous herb with an unpleasant odour.

Part used - Herb.

Therapeutic uses - As an emmenagogue to bring on menstruation. Also an effective nervine.

Prepared as - Infusion.


## Bayberry
MYRICA CERIFERA

Also known as - Candle Berry.

Found wild - United States.

Appearance - Shrub up to 8ft high with shiny leaves and globular berries.

Part used - Bark.

Therapeutic uses - Stimulating and astringent; it improves circulation, and cleanses the stomach and bowels of catarrh. It has a positive effect on the circulatory system of the uterus and is a useful treatment for prolapse of that organ. Also for heavy periods, vaginitis, and simple vaginal discharge.

Prepared as - Powder, fluid extract, tincture, decoction.

### Beth Root
TRILLIUM PENDULUM

Also known as - Woman's Root and Indian Shamrock.

Found wild - North America.

Appearance - Slender herb of low growth with abundant rhizomes emerging from the soil.

Parts used - Rhizome.

Therapeutic uses - To allay excessive menstruation and effective for menorrhagia. Valuable as an astringent and tonic.

Prepared as - Decoction.

### Black Willow Bark
SALIX DISCOLOR

Found wild - United States

Appearance - Typical willow tree.

Parts used - Bark and berries.

Therapeutic uses - Extraordinary powers to lessen sexual libido. Effective for controlling night emissions and premature ejaculations.

Prepared as - Decoction.

### Blue Cohosh
CAULOPHYLLUM THALICTROIDES

Also known as - Squaw root.

Where found - Near streams and swamps in United States.

Appearance - Perennial plant with yellowish green flowers.

Part used - Root.

Therapeutic uses - Traditionally used by Red Indian women during childbirth and to treat absence of periods. Useful as an antispasmodic and relaxant for uterine complaints, including painful menstruation and uterine inflammation. Also for ovarian, urinary and vaginal inflammation and thrush. Useful as a tonic at the menopause.

Prepared as - Powder, decoction, infusion, douche, tincture, fluid extract.

### Burdock
ARCTIUM LAPPA

Also known as - Love leaves.

Found wild - Waste ground throughout UK and Europe.

Appearance - A perennial plant growing to about 4ft with large rhubarb shaped leaves, purple flowers and burrs.

Parts used  - Leaves, dried root and fruits

Therapeutic uses – A valuable blood purifier useful in the treatment of skin eruptions, affecting head, neck and face, such as acne, boils, carbuncles and styes; also for common skin diseases, including eczema, psoriasis and dermatitis. As a diuretic it is useful in sciatica, gout and rheumatism as it aids the removal of waste products.
Improves tissue function by action on mucous and serous membranes: a remedy used by medical herbalists in prescriptions for over-relaxed vaginal tissue.

Prepared as - Decoction (of root and fruits), infusion (of leaves) poultice (of leaves), tincture (of  fruits, root and whole herb), fluid extract.


## Cardamom
ELETTARIA CARDAMOMUM

Also known as - Malabar Cardamom.

Found wild - Ceylon and India.

Appearance - Forest plant with large smooth, dark green leaves and small yellowish flowers.

Part used - Fruits, seeds and oil.

Therapeutic uses - An aromatic herb mainly used in the treatment of flatulence and other digestive problems. Cardamom is also reputed to be a sexual tonic. It is often used in aphrodisiac remedies.

Prepared as - Powder, liquid extract, tincture, essential oil.

## Cascara Sagrada
RHAMNUS PURSHIANA

Also known as - Cascara.

Found wild - North America.

Appearance - A small, low growing tree.

Part used - Bark.

Therapeutic uses - Regarded as one of the safest and purest tonic laxatives.

Prepared as - Decoction. (Reduced dosages used.)

## Celery
APIUM GRAVEOLENS

Found wild - Europe.

Appearance - This is the familiar vegetable.

Parts used - Stem and seeds.

Therapeutic uses - Regarded as one of the most effective herbal aphrodisiacs. It is also a tonic, diuretic and carminative and a most beneficial aid for the relief of rheumatoid troubles.

Prepared as - Decoction from stems or powder (from seeds).

### Centaury
CENFAURIUM ERITHRAEA

Also known as - Feverwort.

Found wild - UK and Europe.

Appearance - Small pink-flowered herb.

Part used - Leaves.

Therapeutic uses - Stomachic, aromatic, bitter. For stomach upsets and anorexia nervosa.

Prepared as - Infusion.

### Chamomile, Belgian
ANFHEMIS NOBILIS

Found wild - Belgium and France (also widely cultivated).

Appearance - A low growing, scented herb with double flowers.

Part used - Flowers.

Therapeutic uses - One of the best remedies for women suffering from nervous upsets and regarded as one of the most reliable tonics. Also used as a stomachic and antispasmodic.

Prepared as - Infusion.

### Clary
SALVIA SCLAREA

Also known as - Christ's Eye and Clary Sage.

Found wild - Common garden plant.

Appearance - Similar to common sage with blue or white flowers.

Part used - Herb, seeds and oil.

Therapeutic uses - It is mainly used for digestive problems. It has antispasmodic properties which are useful in colic and painful menstruation. The old herbalists used it for ophthalmic conditions (clary eye = clear eye). The oil is intoxicating, which may have led to it being regarded as an aphrodisiac. It has been used as a sexual tonic in impotence and as a remedy for postnatal depression.

Prepared as - Infusion, mucilage and oil. The oil should be used only under medical supervision.

### Cotton Root
GOSSYPIUM HERBACEUM

Found wild - Mediterranean islands and the United States.

Appearance - The bark is used medicinally, and is sold in thin strips rolled in twists.

Part used - Bark.

Therapeutic uses - Of great value in the treatment of women's disorders. It contracts the uterus and promotes the menstrual flow. It also aids women whose sexual drive is low.

Prepared as - Infusion

### Damiana
TURNERA DIFFUSA

Found wild - Southern United States and Mexico.

Appearance - Medium-sized shrub.

Parts used - Leaves and stem.

Therapeutic uses - Famous for its aphrodisiac qualities. Also used as a tonic for the aged and those suffering from exhaustion and debility

Prepared as - Infusion.

## Deer's Tongue
LIATRIS ODORATISSIMA

Also known as - America Wild Vanilla.

Found wild - United States.

Appearance - A strong-growing climbing plant.

Parts used Leaves.

Therapeutic uses - A powerful stimulant regarded by the North American Indians as an aphrodisiac. Also a most effective diuretic.

Prepared as - Infusion.

## False Unicorn Root
CHAMAELIRIUM LUTEUM

Also known as -Helonias.

Found wild - Moist habitats in United States.

Appearance -Perennial herb with small greenish-white flowers.

Part used - Rhizome.

Therapeutic uses - Often used in combination with other remedies for spermatorrhoea and impotence. Reproductive tonic in infertility, genito-urinary weaknesses such as prolapse, and laxity of vaginal tissue. Improves ovarian function. Used to treat heavy periods, and simple vaginal discharge. Also indicated as a tonic during the menopause.

Prepared as - Fluid extract, tincture. Small doses only are used. Large doses are emetic.

## Fringetree
CHIONANTHUS VIRGINICA

Found wild - Southern United States.

Appearance - A small tree with inconspicuous white flowers. Has a very bitter taste.

Part used - Bark of the root.

Therapeutic uses -Tonic, alterative and diuretic. Also for treatment of liver disorders, gallstones and jaundice.

Prepared as - Decoction.

## Gentian
GENRIANA LUTEA

Found wild - Alpine meadows.

Appearance - A plant with oblong, pale green leaves and large, yellow scented flowers.

Part used - Root.

Therapeutic use - Regarded as one of the best tonics known.

Prepared as - Decoction and powder.

### Ginger
ZINGIBER OFFICINALE

Found wild - West Indies and China.

Appearance - About one metre high with glossy, aromatic leaves. Its fleshy roots are dried and peeled.

Part used - Rhizome.

Therapeutic uses - Justly famed for its stimulative and carminative properties, and also used as an expectorant. Aids digestion and promotes feeling of warmth and well being.

Prepared as - Powder or decoction.

### Ginseng
PANAX QUINQUEFOLIUM

Also known as - Chinese Panacea, Panax and The Gift of the Gods.

Found wild - China and Mongolia.

Appearance - An erect-growing herb with vivid fleshy leaves and greenish-white
flowers.

Part used - Root.

Therapeutic uses - Recorded prior to 2000 BC, it has properties as an effective herbal aphrodisiac without irritative after effects. Most effective as a tonic for the aged and senile and for digestive troubles. Also assists the central nervous system.

Prepared as Powder or decoction.


## Hydrocotyle
HYDROCOTYLE ASIATICA

Also known as - Indian Pennywort.

Found wild - Tropical India and Africa.

Appearance - A small plant similar to Angelica.

Part used - Leaves.

Therapeutic uses - Claimed in India as an effective herbal aphrodisiac for the middle aged, it is wholesome and safe to use. Also beneficial for treatment of urinary disorders.

Prepared as - Infusion.

## Juniper
JUNIPERUS COMMUNIS

Also known as - Genevrier.

Found wild - Grows in many parts of the world.

Appearance - A coniferous tree.

Part used - Berries, wood, oil.

Therapeutic uses - A stimulating diuretic and carminative usually used in combination with other remedies for short-term treatment of urinary tract diseases. The older herbalists noted that it helped to make childbirth easier. The oil is extremely powerful and must be used in dilution as it can irritate the kidneys and urinary organs. It is reputed to have aphrodisiac properties, resembling cantharides and, if given in overdose, may cause priapism.

Prepared as - Infusion, tincture, oil (to be used only under medical supervision).

## Kava Kava
PIPER METHYSTICUM

Also known as - Intoxicating Pepper.

Found wild - South Sea Islands.

Appearance - Large flowering shrub.

Part used - Root.

Therapeutic uses - Small doses used in combination with other remedies as a tonic in the short-term treatment of ailments of the genito-urinary tract; benign enlarged prostate, nocturnal incontinence; vaginitis; vaginal discharge. Large doses cause inflammation.

Prepared as - Fluid extract, powder. Used in herbal tablets.

### Kola
COLA VERA

Also known as - Kola Nut and Cola Nut.

Found wild - West Africa.

Appearance - A large tree of outstanding elegance.

Part used - Seeds.

Therapeutic uses - Celebrated for its aphrodisiac powers, it is also a nerve stimulant and heart tonic.

Prepared as - Powder.


### Lady's Slipper
CYPRIPEDIUM PUBESCENS

Also known as - Nerve Root.

Found wild - Europe and the United States, but is now an endangered species.

Appearance - A delicate wild orchid.

Part used - Rhizome.

Therapeutic uses - A most effective nervine, used to allay disorders of a nervous origin, including emotional tension and hysteria. It helps to induce natural sleep. It is also antispasmodic and relaxing. A useful treatment for menopausal problems, anxiety states, spontaneous seminal emissions, excessive sexual desire, painful periods.

Prepared as - Powder, decoction, fluid extract, tincture.

## Motherwort
LEONURUS CARDIACA

Found wild - A common garden plant in Britain and northern Europe.

Appearance - A pink-flowered herb of handsome appearance.

Part used Herb.

Therapeutic uses - One of the finest of all nerviness especially for women's troubles. Fine tonic for sufferers from heart disease and a stimulant to the aged.

Prepared as - Infusion.

## MuiraPuama

LIRIOSMA OVATA

Found wild - Brazil.

Appearance - A tree of considerable size.

Part used - Roots.

Therapeutic uses - One of the strongest and most reliable herbal aphrodisiacs known, but not readily available in Britain at present. Can help prolong virility. Also of value to women suffering from nervous exhaustion and debility. A stimulant of extraordinary quality.

Prepared as -Decoction.

### Muskseed
HIBISCUS ABELMOSCHUS

Found wild -India.

Appearance - Small shrub of bold appearance. Both taste and smell are musky.

Part used - Seeds.

Therapeutic uses - An insecticide used since ancient times for ridding the body of lice and scabies.

Prepared as Powder (for external use).

### Oak
QUERCUS ROBUR

Found wild - In most temperate parts of the world.

Appearance - The massive tree which epitomizes the English character.

Part used - Bark.

Therapeutic uses - The oak has tonic properties but is usually prescribed for its astringent qualities. Relieves diarrhoea and dysentery. Used as a gargle it is good for sore throats.

Prepared as - Decoction.

## Oats
AVENA SATIVA

Found wild - In most temperate climates.

Appearance - A common farm crop similar to wheat.

Part used - Seeds.

Therapeutic uses - Helpful as tonic in spermatorrhoea and for menopausal difficulties.

Prepared as - Decoction.

## Paraguay Tea
FLEX PARAGUENSFS

Also known as - Mate Tea.

Found wild - South America.

Appearance - A dense shrub.

Part used - Leaves.

Therapeutic uses- The caffeine content is high and it has excellent stimulant properties. Frequently used as an aphrodisiac and more generally to relieve rheumatism and arthritis.

Prepared as - Infusion.

## Pennyroyal
MENTHA PULEGfUM

Found wild Europe.

Appearance A small herb with a dainty and elegant appearance. It is low growing with tiny leaves and lavender flowers.

Parts used - Leaves and oil.

Therapeutic uses - Chiefly used for its emmenagogue qualities. Known to be the best treatment for obstructed menstruation. Also a gentle stimulant and diaphoretic.

Prepared as - Infusion.

Caution: not to be used during pregnancy.


## Peruvian Bark
CINCHONA OFFFCINALFS

Also known as - Jesuits Bark.

Found wild - The Andes, but cultivated in India and Java.

Appearance - Evergreen tree.

Part used Bark.

Therapeutic uses - Traditionally used for the treatment of fever, and as a gargle for throat conditions, but also useful as a general tonic in debility. Small doses are included in compound remedies for sexual impotence. Correct dosage important. Overuse causes headaches and giddiness.

Prepared as -  Fluid extract, decoction, powder.

## Popular
POPULUS TREMULOIDES

Found wild - Throughout Europe.

Appearance - A very common tree of much elegance.

Part used Bark.

Therapeutic uses Prescribed for its diuretic qualities. Also as a reliable tonic stimulant. Said to be good for treatment of debility. .

Prepared as Decoction.

## Prickly Ash
XANTHOXYLUM AMERICANUM

Also known as- Toothache Tree.

Found wild - Canada and United States.

Appearance - Small tree with prickles on the branches.

Parts used - Berries and root-bark.

Therapeutic uses - Stimulating tonic. Used in arthritis, skin diseases and other conditions where a stimulant is indicated. It is included in traditional remedies for sexual impotence.

Prepared as - Fluid extract, tincture, decoction, powder.

## Pyrethrum
CHRYSANTHEMUM CINERAR1AEFOLIUM

Also known as - Insect flowers.

Found wild - Yugoslavia and the Far East.
Appearance - A feathery-leaved plant about 60 cm (2 feet) high with pink or white daisy-like flowers.
Part used - Flowers.
Therapeutic uses - As an insecticide. Powder is not dangerous to man and is much used for the control of insects, lice, etc.
Prepared as - Powder (for external use).

## Raspberry
RUBUS IDAEUS

Where found - Commonly cultivated in most temperate climates.

Appearance - A bush producing edible fruit.

Part used - Leaves.

Therapeutic uses - Astringent and stimulant. Useful in the treatment of painful periods, easier childbirth, and also as a gargle for sore throat.

Prepared as - Infusion.

## Rosemary
ROSMARINUS OFFICINALIS

Found wild Southern Europe and the Near East.

Appearance A hardy evergreen shrub with fragrant needle-like leaves and tiny blue flowers

Part used - Leaves.

Therapeutic uses - A satisfying nervine, good for persistent headaches and migraine. Known for promoting hair growth.

Prepared as - Infusion.

.

### St John's Wort
HYPERICUM PERFORATUM

Also known as - Hypericum.

Found wild - Europe.

Appearance - A small shrub with bright yellow flowers and black-spotted leaves.

Part used - Leaves.

Therapeutic uses - Menopausal neurosis.

Prepared as - Decoction.

### Saw Palmetto
SERENOA SERRUIATA

Also known as - Sabal.

Found wild - Pacific coast and North America.

Appearance - A palm tree of medium growth.

Part used Barries.

Therapeutic uses - Known to be one of the most effective herbal aphrodisiacs, it is said to preserve virility into old age. It is without irritant effects. It is also a sedative and diuretic.

Prepared as - Infusion.

## Scullcap
SCUTELLARIA LATERIFOLIA

Found wild - United States.

Appearance - A herb of insignificant appearance with pale blue flowers.

Part used - Herb.

Therapeutic uses - Famous as a nervine and tonic, it relieves nervous tension and tremor.

Prepared as - Infusion.

## Squaw Vine
MITCHELLA REP ENS

Also known as - Winter Clover.

Found wild - United States.

Appearance - A small herb of spreading habit.

Parts used - Leaves.

Therapeutic uses - Relieves menstrual problems such as painful and profuse periods, and amenorrhoea. Improves blood supply to the uterus. It is a diuretic and astringent, influencing kidneys, stomach and bowels and stimulating to the nervous system. Used to facilitate childbirth. Also indicated in spermatorrhoea and simple vaginal discharge. Usually combined with other remedies.

Prepared as - Infusion, decoction, douche, fluid extract, tincture.

## Storax
LIQUIDAMBAR ORIENTALIS

Also known as - Sweet Gum.

Found wild - Turkey.

Appearance A small sturdy tree.

Part used Balsam.

Therapeutic uses - One of the best expectorants and a powerful stimulant of value for its aphrodisiac qualities.

Prepared as Balsam.

## Sumbul
FERUIA SUMBUL

Also known as - Musk Root.

Found wild - East Asia.

Appearance-  A shrub of moderate growth.

Parts used - Root.

Therapeutic uses Aneffective nerve stimulant and tonic. Also used as a tonic and antispasmodic.

Prepared as Decoction.

### True Unicorn Root
ALETRIS FARINOSA

Also known as - Colic root.

Found wild - Wet land in United States.

Appearance - Low-growing perennial herb with white bell-shaped flowers.

Part used - Dried rhizome.

Therapeutic uses - Tonic for female generative system, indicated in menstrual problems, such as absence of periods, heavy periods, and prevention of miscarriage. Also used in the treatment of loss of libido and infertility, and as a menopausal tonic.

Prepared as - Powder, tincture, fluid extract. Small doses only. Large does may cause nausea and dizziness.

### Valerian
VALERIANA OFFICINALIS

Found wild Britain in marshy areas.

Appearance - A herb with dark green serrated leaves and lavender-pink flowers. It can grow up to 1.5 metres (5 feet).

Part used Rhizome.

Therapeutic uses - A nervine of extraordinary virtues. Effective for relieving nervous tension or nervous debility and excellent when used as a soporific. One of the best anodynes.

Prepared as - Infusion.

## Veroain
VERBENA OFFICINALIS

Found wild  -Britain.

Appearance  -A roadside herb with heavily toothed leaves and long lilac flowers.

Part used  -Leaves.

Therapeutic uses  -A fine nervine which also relieves depression and anxiety neurosis. Also an emetic and a sudorific.

Prepared as - Infusion.

## Wild Yam
DIOSCORFA VILLOSA

Also known as - Colic Root.

Where found - Tropical countries, United States and Canada.

Appearance - A perennial climbing plant.

Part used - Root.

Therapeutic uses - An antispasmodic useful for neuralgia, colic, flatulence, nausea of pregnancy, spasmodic asthma, cramping pains, painful periods, uterine pain, and rheumatism arising from liver and digestive disorders.

Prepared as - Fluid extract, tincture (the dried root quickly loses its therapeutic potency).

## VITAMINS AND MINERALS

Medical herbalists often prescribe vitamins and minerals to their patients when indicated. Among those that might be helpful for the conditions dealt with in this book are:

### VITAMINB6

A deficiency of vitamin B6 (pyridoxine) is one of the commoner causes of impotency in men and absence of periods in women. it is also related to mental stability. The vitamin is often combined or co-prescribed with zinc.

### VITAMIN E

A fat soluble vitamin discovered in the 1920s, vitamin E is one of the most popular food supplements taken on a regular basis. It is used by the food industry as a natural preservative to give products extra shelf life. As anti-oxidant it slows down the rate at which foods turn rancid. It is found naturally in vegetable oils, such as sunflower oil, peanut oil and wheatgerm oil, and in sunflower seeds, green leafy vegetables, milk, eggs, nuts, wheatgerm, lettuce and soya. The vitamin is available in several different forms, but capsules are the most commonly prescribed. It has a high reputation as an aid to fertility. This is based on the fact that animals, deficient in vitamin E do not have successful pregnancies and that horses given Vitamin E are more fertile.

It was thought that giving vitamin E to women who experience spontaneous abortions might be useful. But this therapy has not been found to be effective. However, the chemical name for the vitamin is tocopherol which is a combination of two Greek words meaning 'I bring childbirth'. There is obviously more work to be done in this area.

## ZINC

This mineral is used in the body for the production of sperm and ova. High concentrations are also found in prostate tissue, prostatic fluid, skin, hair and nails. A deficiency is associated not only with skin diseases, in both men and women, but also with sexual potency, fertility, and absence of periods. Zinc is involved in growth and is a factor in the sexual organs developing to the full size. Girls who are zinc deficient may be late in starting their periods, or the periods may be irregular. Men excrete zinc from the body at each ejaculation, and this may be why over-indulgence in sex can reduce potency in men who do not absorb zinc well, or whose diet is deficient in this mineral. Women are not at risk of losing zinc through their secretions, but may have difficulty in absorbing the mineral. Zinc is also used by the immune system as a defence against infection, and reserves may be reduced to critical levels during a severe illness.

While processed foods may be lacking in zinc, because farmers do not usually add the mineral to the soil, herbs collected from the wild and vegetables grown organically have adequate levels because the zinc is continually recycled. Some herbs used for fertility may indeed contain higher levels of organic zinc. The best food sources are: oysters, herrings, cow's milk, oatmeal, wheatgerm, wheatbran, meats - such as pork and beef - peas, carrots and nuts. The mineral is also available in tablet form and drops. A diet too high in fibre may block the body's absorption of zinc. It is also blocked by tea drinking and excreted by coffee, alcohol and other diuretics.

# Chapter 10

## Seeking professional help

Although this book is aimed at giving those with sexual problems information and guidance on treatment with herbal medicines, it cannot be stressed too much that quicker results can often be achieved by consulting a fully qualified herbal practitioner.

Patients are seen by appointment and in confidence in the practitioner's consulting rooms. Herbal practitioners qualified with the National Institute of Medical Herbalist (recognised by the initials MNIMH or FNIMH after their names) are trained to deal with a wide range of medical problems, although some practitioners may specialise in certain medical areas.

The Institute, founded in 1864, is the oldest established body of practising medical herbalists in the world. Members can be found in most towns in the US and UK.

Currently, there are 17 U.S. states, and five Canadian provinces, the District of Columbia and the U.S. territories of Puerto Rico and the U.S. Virgin Islands require licensing for naturopathic doctors. For graduates of the herbalism school, there is no real specific federal- or state-level of regulation. However, if you work as a chiropractor or another health practitioner, you may have to meet some licensing requirements for that particular field in order to practice. Membership to the American Herbalists Guild can grant an additional degree of professionalism, since guild members are required to complete a set of standardized educational requirements.
The aim of herbal medicine is not just to relieve symptoms but to offer the sufferer an increased level of general health. The practitioner takes an holistic approach to his patients, an approach that is being followed more and more by other primary health care and complementary medicine practitioners.

He will, therefore, take into account not only physical symptoms but also any mental stress or emotional problems which may be relevant. Both the body and the mind conform to the laws of nature, one of the most important of which is the law of homoeostasis - the ability of the individual to be self-regulating, despite changes in the environment. It is the law of balance that has enabled us to survive for thousands of years despite changes, or threats, in the environment, whether it be a simple change in temperature, or an infection due to pathogenic microorganisms. The same law also applies to the mind, which attempts to maintain a healthy equilibrium in the face of external stresses. Disease is produced when outside threats, or changes, are too overwhelming and the individual fails to respond or adapt healthily.

Many sexual and relationship problems can be traced back to imbalances in the individual's early family life - dominant mother and weak fathers, or aggressive fathers and timid mothers; rivalry for attention among children in large families, or the child's loss of nurturing due to both parents working; devaluing or abuse of children by parents; one parent constantly belittling the other; and the modern phenomenon - children of single parents – single by choice rather than from war or other natural calamity.

Sadly, it is such a common occurrence today. And what an explosion of problems we are now seeing and will see due to this and similar problems such as adopted children angry at the loss of their natural mothers. Nature demands balance. There is always a price to pay, always a compensation, for imbalance. The mind as well as the body pays by becoming ill.

It is not always easy to treat oneself appropriately. It quite often needs a trained practitioner to give guidance so that the deeper reasons for an illness and not just the superficial are treated.

# Glossary of common medical terms

Very often when reading, or on having a medical consultation, medical terms are used which may not be familiar. This short list will help to make some of the more common ones a little clearer.

Alterative -Any substance that can beneficially alter the condition of a patient.

Amenorrhoea -Cessation of the menstrual flow.

Anodyne -Any substance which eases pain.

Antiseptic -Any substance that prevents putrefaction.

Antispasmodic -Any substance that prevents or relieves spasms.

Anthelmintic -Any herb acting against intestinal worms.

Aperient -Any substance producing the natural evacuation of the bowels.

Aphrodisiac -Any substance that stimulates sexual functions.

Astringent -Any substance which causes contraction of body tissues.

Cardiac -Any condition affecting or pertaining to the heart.

Carminative -Any substance that relieves pain caused by flatulence.

Corrective -Any substance that restores normal conditions.

Debility -Feebleness of health.

Degenerative -Deterioration or change in tissue structure.

Demulcent -Any soothing medicine.

Deobstruent -Any substance that frees the natural orifices of the body.

Diaphoretic -Any substance inducing perspiration.

Diuretic -Any substance that increases the flow of urine.

Dysmenorrhoea -Excessive pain during menstruation.

Emetic -Any substance that causes vomiting.

Emmenagogue -Any drug that stimulates menstruation.

Emollient -Any substance that soothes and lubricates.

Frigidity -An inability on the part of a woman to reach orgasm.

Haemostatic -Any substance that checks bleeding and aids the clotting of blood.

Homosexual -A sexual attraction between persons of the same sex.

Impotency -An inability on the part of a man to achieve sexual intercourse.

Insecticide -Any substance that is fatal to insects.

Laxative-Any substance that induces gentle, easy bowel action.

Leucorrhoea -Any mucus discharge from female genitals.

Libido -Sex drive.

Masturbation -Manual stimulation to obtain an orgasm.

Menorrhagia -Excessive flow in menstruation.

Narcotic -Any drug that induces stupor and insensibility.

Nephritis -Any drug that affects the kidneys.

Nervine -Any substance that restores the nerves to a normal tone.

Oxytocic -Any drug that contracts the uterus and hastens childbirth.

Parturient -Any product used during childbirth.

Resolvent -Any substance that reduces swelling.

Sedative -Any substance used to placate 'nerves'.

Soporific -Any substance used to promote sleep.

Ppermatorrhoea -Passing of semen without orgasm or erection.

Stimulant -Any substance used to promote the reserve power of the body and produce strength and energy.

Stomachic -Any substance that allays stomach disorders.

Sudorific -Any substance producing heavy perspiration.

Tonic -Any substance that, if used regularly, will promote vivacity and well being.

**Vaginismus** -Spasmodic contractions of the entrance of the vagina on attempted intercourse.

**Vaginitis** -Inflammation of the vagina.